KETO DIET

MEAL PLANNER

....

Healthy Mind Comes
From
Healthy Body

December

Week 1   12-31-18 to 01-06-19

○ 31. MONDAY

PRIORITIES

○ 1. TUESDAY

○ 2. WEDNESDAY

GOALS & ACHIEVEMENTS

○ 3. THURSDAY

○ 4. FRIDAY

○ 5. SATURDAY / 6. SUNDAY

January

Week 2

01-07-19 to 01-13-19

○ 7. MONDAY

PRIORITIES

○ 8. TUESDAY

○ 9. WEDNESDAY

GOALS & ACHIEVEMENTS

○ 10. THURSDAY

○ 11. FRIDAY

○ 12. SATURDAY / 13. SUNDAY

January

Week 3   01-14-19 to 01-20-19

○ 14. MONDAY

PRIORITIES

○ 15. TUESDAY

○ 16. WEDNESDAY

GOALS & ACHIEVEMENTS

○ 17. THURSDAY

○ 18. FRIDAY

○ 19. SATURDAY / 20. SUNDAY

January

Week 4   01-21-19 to 01-27-19

○ 21. MONDAY

PRIORITIES

○ 22. TUESDAY

○ 23. WEDNESDAY

GOALS & ACHIEVEMENTS

○ 24. THURSDAY

○ 25. FRIDAY

○ 26. SATURDAY / 27. SUNDAY

January

Week 5   01-28-19 to 02-03-19

○ 28. MONDAY

PRIORITIES

○ 29. TUESDAY

○ 30. WEDNESDAY

GOALS & ACHIEVEMENTS

○ 31. THURSDAY

○ 1. FRIDAY

○ 2. SATURDAY / 3. SUNDAY

Monthly Achievements

February

Week 6

02-04-19 to 02-10-19

○ 4. MONDAY

PRIORITIES

○ 5. TUESDAY

○ 6. WEDNESDAY

GOALS & ACHIEVEMENTS

○ 7. THURSDAY

○ 8. FRIDAY

○ 9. SATURDAY / 10. SUNDAY

February

Week 7   02-11-19 to 02-17-19

○ 11. MONDAY

PRIORITIES

○ 12. TUESDAY

○ 13. WEDNESDAY

GOALS & ACHIEVEMENTS

○ 14. THURSDAY

○ 15. FRIDAY

○ 16. SATURDAY / 17. SUNDAY

February

Week 8   02-18-19 to 02-24-19

○ 18. MONDAY

PRIORITIES

○ 19. TUESDAY

○ 20. WEDNESDAY

GOALS & ACHIEVEMENTS

○ 21. THURSDAY

○ 22. FRIDAY

○ 23. SATURDAY / 24. SUNDAY

February

Week 9   02-25-19 to 03-03-19

○ 25. MONDAY

PRIORITIES

○ 26. TUESDAY

○ 27. WEDNESDAY

GOALS & ACHIEVEMENTS

○ 28. THURSDAY

○ 1. FRIDAY

○ 2. SATURDAY / 3. SUNDAY

Monthly Achievements

March

Week 10   03-04-19 to 03-10-19

○ 4. MONDAY

PRIORITIES

○ 5. TUESDAY

○ 6. WEDNESDAY

GOALS & ACHIEVEMENTS

○ 7. THURSDAY

○ 8. FRIDAY

○ 9. SATURDAY / 10. SUNDAY

March

Week 11   03-11-19 to 03-17-19

○ 11. MONDAY

PRIORITIES

○ 12. TUESDAY

○ 13. WEDNESDAY

GOALS & ACHIEVEMENTS

○ 14. THURSDAY

○ 15. FRIDAY

○ 16. SATURDAY / 17. SUNDAY

March

Week 12   03-18-19 to 03-24-19

○ 18. MONDAY

PRIORITIES

○ 19. TUESDAY

○ 20. WEDNESDAY

GOALS & ACHIEVEMENTS

○ 21. THURSDAY

○ 22. FRIDAY

○ 23. SATURDAY / 24. SUNDAY

March

Week 13   03-25-19 to 03-31-19

○ 25. MONDAY

PRIORITIES

○ 26. TUESDAY

○ 27. WEDNESDAY

GOALS & ACHIEVEMENTS

○ 28. THURSDAY

○ 29. FRIDAY

○ 30. SATURDAY / 31. SUNDAY

Monthly Achievements

April

Week 14

04-01-19 to 04-07-19

○ 1. MONDAY

PRIORITIES

○ 2. TUESDAY

○ 3. WEDNESDAY

GOALS & ACHIEVEMENTS

○ 4. THURSDAY

○ 5. FRIDAY

○ 6. SATURDAY / 7. SUNDAY

April

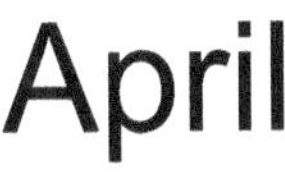

Week 15

04-08-19 to 04-14-19

○ 8. MONDAY

PRIORITIES

○ 9. TUESDAY

○ 10. WEDNESDAY

GOALS & ACHIEVEMENTS

○ 11. THURSDAY

○ 12. FRIDAY

○ 13. SATURDAY / 14. SUNDAY

April
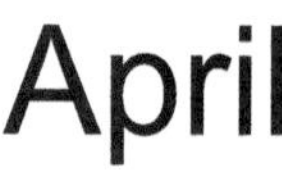

Week 16

04-15-19 to 04-21-19

○ 15. MONDAY

PRIORITIES

○ 16. TUESDAY

○ 17. WEDNESDAY

GOALS & ACHIEVEMENTS

○ 18. THURSDAY

○ 19. FRIDAY

○ 20. SATURDAY / 21. SUNDAY

April

Week 17

04-22-19 to 04-28-19

○ 22. MONDAY

PRIORITIES

○ 23. TUESDAY

○ 24. WEDNESDAY

GOALS & ACHIEVEMENTS

○ 25. THURSDAY

○ 26. FRIDAY

○ 27. SATURDAY / 28. SUNDAY

April

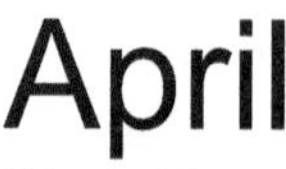

Week 18

04-29-19 to 05-05-19

○ 29. MONDAY

PRIORITIES

○ 30. TUESDAY

○ 1. WEDNESDAY

GOALS & ACHIEVEMENTS

○ 2. THURSDAY

○ 3. FRIDAY

○ 4. SATURDAY / 5. SUNDAY

Monthly Achievements

May

05-06-19 to 05-12-19

○ 6. MONDAY

PRIORITIES

○ 7. TUESDAY

○ 8. WEDNESDAY

GOALS & ACHIEVEMENTS

○ 9. THURSDAY

○ 10. FRIDAY

○ 11. SATURDAY / 12. SUNDAY

May

Week 20

05-13-19 to 05-19-19

○ 13. MONDAY

PRIORITIES

○ 14. TUESDAY

○ 15. WEDNESDAY

GOALS & ACHIEVEMENTS

○ 16. THURSDAY

○ 17. FRIDAY

○ 18. SATURDAY / 19. SUNDAY

May

Week 21

05-20-19 to 05-26-19

○ 20. MONDAY

PRIORITIES

○ 21. TUESDAY

○ 22. WEDNESDAY

GOALS & ACHIEVEMENTS

○ 23. THURSDAY

○ 24. FRIDAY

○ 25. SATURDAY / 26. SUNDAY

May

Week 22

05-27-19 to 06-02-19

○ 27. MONDAY

PRIORITIES

○ 28. TUESDAY

○ 29. WEDNESDAY

GOALS & ACHIEVEMENTS

○ 30. THURSDAY

○ 31. FRIDAY

○ 1. SATURDAY / 2. SUNDAY

Monthly Achievements

June

○ 3. MONDAY

PRIORITIES

○ 4. TUESDAY

○ 5. WEDNESDAY

GOALS & ACHIEVEMENTS

○ 6. THURSDAY

○ 7. FRIDAY

○ 8. SATURDAY / 9. SUNDAY

June

Week 24   06-10-19 to 06-16-19

○ 10. MONDAY

PRIORITIES

○ 11. TUESDAY

○ 12. WEDNESDAY

GOALS & ACHIEVEMENTS

○ 13. THURSDAY

○ 14. FRIDAY

○ 15. SATURDAY / 16. SUNDAY

June

Week 25

06-17-19 to 06-23-19

○ 17. MONDAY

PRIORITIES

○ 18. TUESDAY

○ 19. WEDNESDAY

GOALS & ACHIEVEMENTS

○ 20. THURSDAY

○ 21. FRIDAY

○ 22. SATURDAY / 23. SUNDAY

June

Week 26   06-24-19 to 06-30-19

○ 24. MONDAY

PRIORITIES

○ 25. TUESDAY

○ 26. WEDNESDAY

GOALS & ACHIEVEMENTS

○ 27. THURSDAY

○ 28. FRIDAY

○ 29. SATURDAY / 30. SUNDAY

Monthly Achievements

July
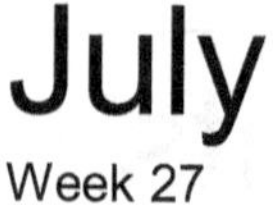

Week 27

07-01-19 to 07-07-19

○ 1. MONDAY

PRIORITIES

○ 2. TUESDAY

○ 3. WEDNESDAY

GOALS & ACHIEVEMENTS

○ 4. THURSDAY

○ 5. FRIDAY

○ 6. SATURDAY / 7. SUNDAY

July

Week 28

07-08-19 to 07-14-19

○ 8. MONDAY

PRIORITIES

○ 9. TUESDAY

○ 10. WEDNESDAY

GOALS & ACHIEVEMENTS

○ 11. THURSDAY

○ 12. FRIDAY

○ 13. SATURDAY / 14. SUNDAY

July

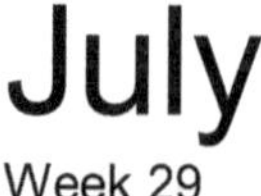

Week 29

07-15-19 to 07-21-19

○ 15. MONDAY

PRIORITIES

○ 16. TUESDAY

○ 17. WEDNESDAY

GOALS & ACHIEVEMENTS

○ 18. THURSDAY

○ 19. FRIDAY

○ 20. SATURDAY / 21. SUNDAY

July

Week 30

07-22-19 to 07-28-19

○ 22. MONDAY

PRIORITIES

○ 23. TUESDAY

○ 24. WEDNESDAY

GOALS & ACHIEVEMENTS

○ 25. THURSDAY

○ 26. FRIDAY

○ 27. SATURDAY / 28. SUNDAY

July

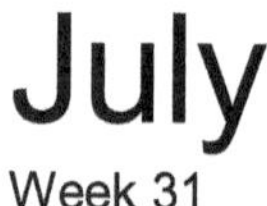

Week 31

07-29-19 to 08-04-19

○ 29. MONDAY

PRIORITIES

○ 30. TUESDAY

○ 31. WEDNESDAY

GOALS & ACHIEVEMENTS

○ 1. THURSDAY

○ 2. FRIDAY

○ 3. SATURDAY / 4. SUNDAY

Monthly Achievements

August

Week 32   08-05-19 to 08-11-19

○ 5. MONDAY

PRIORITIES

○ 6. TUESDAY

○ 7. WEDNESDAY

GOALS & ACHIEVEMENTS

○ 8. THURSDAY

○ 9. FRIDAY

○ 10. SATURDAY / 11. SUNDAY

August

Week 33   08-12-19 to 08-18-19

○ 12. MONDAY

PRIORITIES

○ 13. TUESDAY

○ 14. WEDNESDAY

GOALS & ACHIEVEMENTS

○ 15. THURSDAY

○ 16. FRIDAY

○ 17. SATURDAY / 18. SUNDAY

August

Week 34

08-19-19 to 08-25-19

○ 19. MONDAY

PRIORITIES

○ 20. TUESDAY

○ 21. WEDNESDAY

GOALS & ACHIEVEMENTS

○ 22. THURSDAY

○ 23. FRIDAY

○ 24. SATURDAY / 25. SUNDAY

August

Week 35   08-26-19 to 09-01-19

○ 26. MONDAY

PRIORITIES

○ 27. TUESDAY

○ 28. WEDNESDAY

GOALS & ACHIEVEMENTS

○ 29. THURSDAY

○ 30. FRIDAY

○ 31. SATURDAY / 1. SUNDAY

Monthly Achievements

September

Week 36

09-02-19 to 09-08-19

○ 2. MONDAY

PRIORITIES

○ 3. TUESDAY

○ 4. WEDNESDAY

GOALS & ACHIEVEMENTS

○ 5. THURSDAY

○ 6. FRIDAY

○ 7. SATURDAY / 8. SUNDAY

September

Week 37

09-09-19 to 09-15-19

◯ 9. MONDAY

PRIORITIES

◯ 10. TUESDAY

◯ 11. WEDNESDAY

GOALS & ACHIEVEMENTS

◯ 12. THURSDAY

◯ 13. FRIDAY

◯ 14. SATURDAY / 15. SUNDAY

September

Week 38

09-16-19 to 09-22-19

○ 16. MONDAY

PRIORITIES

○ 17. TUESDAY

○ 18. WEDNESDAY

GOALS & ACHIEVEMENTS

○ 19. THURSDAY

○ 20. FRIDAY

○ 21. SATURDAY / 22. SUNDAY

September

Week 39

09-23-19 to 09-29-19

○ 23. MONDAY

PRIORITIES

○ 24. TUESDAY

○ 25. WEDNESDAY

GOALS & ACHIEVEMENTS

○ 26. THURSDAY

○ 27. FRIDAY

○ 28. SATURDAY / 29. SUNDAY

September

Week 40   09-30-19 to 10-06-19

○ 30. MONDAY

PRIORITIES

○ 1. TUESDAY

○ 2. WEDNESDAY

GOALS & ACHIEVEMENTS

○ 3. THURSDAY

○ 4. FRIDAY

○ 5. SATURDAY / 6. SUNDAY

Monthly Achievements

October

○ 7. MONDAY

PRIORITIES

○ 8. TUESDAY

○ 9. WEDNESDAY

GOALS & ACHIEVEMENTS

○ 10. THURSDAY

○ 11. FRIDAY

○ 12. SATURDAY / 13. SUNDAY

October

Week 42

10-14-19 to 10-20-19

○ 14. MONDAY

PRIORITIES

○ 15. TUESDAY

○ 16. WEDNESDAY

GOALS & ACHIEVEMENTS

○ 17. THURSDAY

○ 18. FRIDAY

○ 19. SATURDAY / 20. SUNDAY

October

Week 43

10-21-19 to 10-27-19

○ 21. MONDAY

PRIORITIES

○ 22. TUESDAY

○ 23. WEDNESDAY

GOALS & ACHIEVEMENTS

○ 24. THURSDAY

○ 25. FRIDAY

○ 26. SATURDAY / 27. SUNDAY

October

Week 44   10-28-19 to 11-03-19

⭘ 28. MONDAY

PRIORITIES

⭘ 29. TUESDAY

⭘ 30. WEDNESDAY

GOALS & ACHIEVEMENTS

⭘ 31. THURSDAY

⭘ 1. FRIDAY

⭘ 2. SATURDAY / 3. SUNDAY

Monthly Achievements

November

11-04-19 to 11-10-19

○ 4. MONDAY

PRIORITIES

○ 5. TUESDAY

○ 6. WEDNESDAY

GOALS & ACHIEVEMENTS

○ 7. THURSDAY

○ 8. FRIDAY

○ 9. SATURDAY / 10. SUNDAY

November

Week 46

11-11-19 to 11-17-19

○ 11. MONDAY

PRIORITIES

○ 12. TUESDAY

○ 13. WEDNESDAY

GOALS & ACHIEVEMENTS

○ 14. THURSDAY

○ 15. FRIDAY

○ 16. SATURDAY / 17. SUNDAY

November

Week 47   11-18-19 to 11-24-19

○ 18. MONDAY

PRIORITIES

○ 19. TUESDAY

○ 20. WEDNESDAY

GOALS & ACHIEVEMENTS

○ 21. THURSDAY

○ 22. FRIDAY

○ 23. SATURDAY / 24. SUNDAY

November

11-25-19 to 12-01-19

○ 25. MONDAY

PRIORITIES

○ 26. TUESDAY

○ 27. WEDNESDAY

GOALS & ACHIEVEMENTS

○ 28. THURSDAY

○ 29. FRIDAY

○ 30. SATURDAY / 1. SUNDAY

Monthly Achievements

December

Week 49

12-02-19 to 12-08-19

○ 2. MONDAY

PRIORITIES

○ 3. TUESDAY

○ 4. WEDNESDAY

GOALS & ACHIEVEMENTS

○ 5. THURSDAY

○ 6. FRIDAY

○ 7. SATURDAY / 8. SUNDAY

December

Week 50   12-09-19 to 12-15-19

○ 9. MONDAY

PRIORITIES

○ 10. TUESDAY

○ 11. WEDNESDAY

GOALS & ACHIEVEMENTS

○ 12. THURSDAY

○ 13. FRIDAY

○ 14. SATURDAY / 15. SUNDAY

December

Week 51   12-16-19 to 12-22-19

○ 16. MONDAY

○ 17. TUESDAY

○ 18. WEDNESDAY

GOALS & ACHIEVEMENTS

○ 19. THURSDAY

○ 20. FRIDAY

○ 21. SATURDAY / 22. SUNDAY

December

Week 52   12-23-19 to 12-29-19

○ 23. MONDAY

PRIORITIES

○ 24. TUESDAY

○ 25. WEDNESDAY

GOALS & ACHIEVEMENTS

○ 26. THURSDAY

○ 27. FRIDAY

○ 28. SATURDAY / 29. SUNDAY

December

Week 1   12-30-19 to 01-05-20

○ 30. MONDAY

PRIORITIES

○ 31. TUESDAY

○ 1. WEDNESDAY

GOALS & ACHIEVEMENTS

○ 2. THURSDAY

○ 3. FRIDAY

○ 4. SATURDAY / 5. SUNDAY

www.ingramcontent.com/pod-product-compliance
Lightning Source LLC
Chambersburg PA
CBHW050756240726
48654CB00008B/518